An Anti-Cancer Diet

Prevent & reverse cancer.
Live longer & look younger.
Lower cholesterol & lose weight.

Robert Korczynski

To my mother, Jo Ann Korczynska, who always asks me to write things down, so she can have them to read again another day.

The website **http://www.ananticancerdiet.com** supports this book, and has links to cancer fighting information, recommended products, and Vegan recipes.

Contents

Introduction

This book has been created to empower the reader with the knowledge of how to prevent many types of cancers, and the best diet to follow when recovering from cancer treatment; it is not a replacement for medical treatment from your doctor. This same diet produces the best heart health, cholesterol numbers, and overall body health.

It is, "An Anti-Cancer Diet," because it's consistent with the diet recommended by the American Cancer Society (ACS), that is, a mostly plant-based, or Vegan diet (no meat, dairy, or eggs). In this book you will find healthy sources of essential amino acids, fats that are good for you, and foods that can help you live longer.

In 1999, the American Cancer Society, the American Dietetic Association, the American Academy of Pediatrics, the National Institutes of Health, and the American Heart Association all jointly endorsed and promoted a plant-based diet for optimal health.

The American Cancer Society currently recommends avoiding meat, dairy, and eggs, as much as possible, both for people who are recovering from cancer, as well as for people who have a family history of cancer.

Taking it one step further, all people would benefit from the cancer-preventing qualities of a plant-based, or Vegan diet. This is not saying that if you want to eat a Vegan diet, you have to go, "cold turkey." What about starting out with half your meals Vegan, and then gradually shifting as many meals as possible over to meat, dairy, and egg free?

Soymilk, rice milk, almond milk, hemp milk, and oat milk are available alternatives to cow's milk for cereal, and drinking water is encouraged as a replacement for drinking cow's milk with meals.

Meat substitutes are available in the form of different types of tofu, fresh and frozen, and many different types of mushrooms. Adapting family recipes to make them Vegan is encouraged, and tofu and mushroom options are detailed in separate chapters.

Eleven supplements are also recommended that show the ability to destroy cancer cells, both by switching on a gene that tells cancer cells to die like normal cells, and by switching on another gene that tells a cancer cell to dissolve itself with digestive enzymes; these eleven supplements also balance your body pH, and change your body from the low-oxygen-acidic environment that cancer thrives in, to a neutral to base pH, and oxygenated cells.

Chapter 1:
Foods that are bad for you

If you are recovering from cancer, or cooking for someone who is, then you should probably avoid all forms of animal protein when you prepare food. This includes all meat (pork, beef, chicken, fish, etc.), and all dairy (yogurt, cheese, milk, etc.), as well as eggs; animal proteins make you acidic, and cancers thrive in acidic conditions. Also, avoid high-fructose corn syrup, most sugars, and carbonated beverages.

Avoid hydrogenated and partially hydrogenated oils, or "trans-fats;" they are in most non-dairy creamers, as well as many other packaged items, even some of those labeled, "0 grams of trans fat per serving." If you read the ingredients, hydrogenated oils or partially hydrogenated oils are sometimes in the list. Hydrogenated oils seem to turn on aging genes that, among other things, harden your arteries.

Just to be safe, you may also want to avoid cottonseed oil; it is sometimes used to make potato chips, and other packaged items. Cottonseed oil is accused of multiple problems: 1) they may use pesticides on cotton that cannot be used on standard food crops, 2) since 1996, most cotton grown in the U.S. has been, "genetically modified," and 3) regardless of which pesticides they use, cotton is one of the most chemically intensive crops in the U.S., and pesticides tend to concentrate in the seed oils.

Avoid using microwave ovens to heat anything, including water; they are banned in Russia due to health problems associated with both being around them while they are operating, as well as consuming foods that have been, "micro waved."

The claim is that microwaves form, "radiolytic compounds," in the food; radiolytic compounds are believed to cause cancer and mutations.

Chapter 2:
Foods that are good for you

Lots of different vegetables, fruits, nuts, and a variety of whole grains, peas, beans, hemp seeds, tofu, coconut oil, maple syrup, Kombu (brown seaweed), and blue green algae start the list of foods that are good for you.

Oddly enough, most people spend over half their food budget per month, just on meat, dairy, and eggs! This means that if you are avoiding meat, dairy, and eggs, you can buy organic vegetables and fruits, and soy, rice, almond, hemp, or oat milk with your savings. You can make the main course the exotic mushroom you perfectly seasoned and cooked. It is actually cheaper to eat healthy, than to not eat healthy. You can shop at Trader Joes, and Whole Foods, and other "health food" stores in your area, and it won't cost you more than shopping at a regular store, if you count meat, dairy, and eggs.

Foods that are fresh are the best for you, so farmers markets are a great place to shop, since you get vegetables picked usually that morning, or the night before. Plus you don't have to figure out what is "local, and in season," as many people advise we eat vegetables and fruits that come from the area you are living in, and many people advise eating seasonal fruits and vegetables. If you do have a farmer's market, get to know some vendors, and ask them for suggestions.

Chapter 3:
Hemp the super food

Hemp is an astonishing plant; it has every essential amino acid (protein) as well as every essential fatty acid (fat) that your body needs. It is an all-in-one food source that provides your body with everything it needs to function, and to heal itself.

Hemp seeds are available in Whole Foods, and in some other stores, and consuming just an ounce or two per day provides every amino acid and every fatty acid (Omega 3, 6, 9, etc), your body needs. Thanks to the company, "Nutiva," we can now buy hemp seeds in the United States that are grown in Canada.

A great way to eat them is sprinkled on oatmeal, 3 tablespoons (about 1½ ounces), and that's it for the day! Or try a hemp-banana-smoothie with orange juice, frozen chunks of banana, and 3 tablespoons of hemp seeds; it kind of tastes like an "orange whip." Hemp seeds, sometimes called, "hemp nuts," can also be added to a variety of dishes, or salads. They can also be simply eaten by the handful for a quick snack.

It is possible to lose weight by eating hemp seeds. The logic goes like this, if you give your body all it needs in proteins and fats, your body won't "crave" foods that are bad for you. Less craving means less snacking, and that leads to the pounds coming off.

If you are eating a Vegan diet, the key advantage to hemp seeds is that you don't have to worry about protein combining, or how to cook new foods as a vegetarian, and you don't have to worry about getting enough protein, or anything else, for that matter. If you just eat 3 tablespoons of hemp seeds one to three times a day, you will give your body everything it needs to heal, and to function at its best. Also eat blue green algae, juice organic vegetables, and follow the recommended anti-cancer diet.

Chapter 4:
Sources of good fats

Coconut oil has rare medium-chain saturated fats, shown in all lab studies to be extraordinarily good for you. Other than coconut, this kind of fat is only found in mother's milk; we know that the immune system is built in the first two years in humans, and that babies weaned after the age of two have stronger immune systems. The connection between coconut oil improving immune strength (for fighting cancer) has not been established, but as coconut oil is the only known source of medium chain fats outside of mother's milk, it seems hard to deny that it might be useful. Coconut oil has been shown to lower bad cholesterol, and to have a variety of health benefits.

Other good fats include walnut oil, and hemp seed oil. Walnut and hemp oil have a perfect balance of Omega 3 to Omega 6 fats for the human body (about 2½ parts Omega 6, to 1 part Omega 3), and can be purchased at health food stores nationwide. The difference is that hemp contains the "super" Omega 3 and 6 fats that older people cannot make out of regular Omega 3 and 6 fats; again, hemp is a complete food source, providing all essential fats you need.

With the exception of Flax seed oil that has around 75% Omega 3 fats, all other oils available in the grocery store are basically the same; olive, corn, peanut, soy, sunflower, safflower, canola, and any other type of clear, blond "vegetable" oil, are just different flavors of mostly Omega 6 fats. Canola may have half the "long-chain" (bad) saturated fats of corn or soybean oil, but they all have around 75% Omega 6 fats, which Americans get too much of anyway, and they all contain almost no Omega 3 fats; all vegetable oils have very low amounts of bad fats, compared to any meat, dairy, or eggs.

If you remember back in the 1970's, the U.S. Government recommended eating olive oil to reduce bad cholesterol, and advised avoiding coconut oil. These both appear to be misguided statements.

Olive oil (mostly Omega 6 fats) is only good for your cholesterol numbers if you eat a lot of seafood (mostly Omega 3 fats), as most Italians do. Most Americans do not eat seafood daily, like Italians, and so they never got the health benefits of olive oil. To be clear, olive oil is not particularly good for someone on a Vegan diet, as it is lacking in Omega 3 essential fatty acids; Vegans should stick to hemp, walnut, and coconut oil for health. A nice olive oil is good for vinaigrettes, and as a finishing oil, to add a little flavor to a dish.

Hemp oil has a strong flavor, which is why walnut oil is sometimes a better choice for cooking; walnut oil has a medium smoke point, and still provides balanced Omega 3 to Omega 6 fats. For high heat frying, use peanut oil, as it has the highest smoke point; and for medium high heat frying, try a little walnut oil and peanut oil together.

When coconut oil was tested for its effects on cholesterol in the 1970s, the samples used were "hydrogenated" coconut oil. Hydrogenation is an industrial process for stabilizing oils at room temperature by bubbling hydrogen gas up thru the oil, until some of the hydrogen atoms get stuck in the oil. We now call hydrogenated oils, "trans-fats," and we think that they are 10 times worse than long chain saturated fats, like from meat. Why they didn't test un-hydrogenated coconut oil is a mystery, but we now know that the studies performed on coconut oil in the 1970s revealed that trans-fats are bad for us, *not* coconut oil.

Sadly, they did not follow the, "scientific method." If they were going to test coconut oil, they should have tested pure oil, rather than hydrogenated coconut oil, which is an industrial food product that consumers can't buy at the grocery store. The scientific method would have required three study groups, one group that changed nothing (or took a placebo), a second group that added plain coconut oil to their diet, and a third group that added hydrogenated coconut oil to their diet.

Had they performed the study, "scientifically," we would have known thirty years ago that trans-fats are horrible for us, and that plain coconut oil is extremely good at lowering bad cholesterol. Instead, we had thirty years of misinformation, and increasingly high rates of cholesterol.

If your doctor or nutritionist has told you to avoid avocados, and to eat salmon and chicken for your health, they are sadly misinformed. Avocados are high in plant-based long chain saturated fats that in meat, like fish, or anything else, are bad for you in excess of 20 grams per day. The fats from plants are always better for you than the fats from any meat, fish, dairy, or egg. Some of the fats in avocados may be "long chain saturated fats," but they are not necessarily "bad fats."

Avocados can be eaten in any amount, by anyone, at any time, including Vegans, as they are not going to be getting many long chain saturated fats from animal sources, anyway.

Chapter 5:
Avoid eating sugar

Avoid eating as much sugar as possible, especially avoid high fructose corn syrup, which is so refined that it moves into your bloodstream, and out of your blood stream very quickly, spiking your insulin levels. The opposite of this is, "complex carbohydrates," things like whole grain flourless bread, brown rice, and any other cooked grain are complex carbohydrates; the same as a spoonful of sugar, it just takes your body a couple of hours to get the sugar.

The only sugar recommended is grade B maple syrup, which has liquid minerals, and has been shown (along with lemon juice and cayenne pepper, mixed with water), to provide all the nutrition required for 30 days in a, "cleansing fast," consuming nothing else but filtered water.

The best replacement for sugar is stevia; all other calorie-free sugars are chemicals that may be very bad for you. Stevia is a sweet tasting, naturally occurring substance that we can't digest; it is found in high amounts in bananas, and is available to purchase like sugar as a sugar-replacement for diabetics. Stevia has also been shown to have a whole list of health benefits, and is therefore a great and healthy way to replace sugar in your house.

Another reason to avoid sugar, in general, is that Candita yeast can be living inside you, either along with cancer, or without cancer. Yeasts living inside you love sugar; and avoiding all sugar, including maple syrup, can help starve them out.

Colloidal silver will kill yeasts off if you built up a level of silver in your bloodstream by drinking some everyday, for 10 days. Always follow colloidal silver with a probiotic supplement once a day, starting the day after you finish the silver, and continuing daily for two weeks; this reestablishes the good intestinal bacteria you killed off with the silver.

Chapter 6:
Juicing raw vegetables

There is a general rule in progressive health and nutrition that 70% of your diet should be raw foods. Raw vegetables provide oxygen to your cells, as well as a variety of other compounds. For optimum health, you should either consume a diet made up of 70% raw foods, or juice raw vegetables and fruit everyday. Personally, I think juicing is easier.

The standard carrot/beat/celery is a good all-around juice to start with, but you can add almost anything, the greater the variety, the better. Beet juice fights cancer by increasing oxygen uptake by 400%, and beets contain other active anti-cancer ingredients, like phytonutrients (the bright colors).

From a raw perspective, juicing is a very convenient way to cheat, and still get your "raw" food benefits. Try juicing all the vegetables you can think of; a juice with 6, 8, or 10 vegetables, and a few fruits, is a great way to consume raw nutrients without snacking on vegetables all day long, or eating salads for every meal. Any standard brand juicer will work fine, and it's a great investment of a few hundred dollars.

When you buy vegetables, try to buy organic vegetables for juicing (and for cooking). When you buy fruits, think of how thick the skin is; thick-skinned fruits, like bananas and oranges, are going to be pealed anyway, so it's probably fine to get non-organic; any thin-skinned fruits that you consume or juice, skin and all, should be organic.

When you juice, make each day's juice right before you drink it. Freshly made juice should be consumed within 5 minutes of being made, if possible.

Always follow juice with an equal amount of room temperature, filtered water.

Chapter 7:
Additional Supplements

Vitamin A, all the Vitamin Bs including Vitamin B-12, Vitamin C, Vitamin D, and Vitamin E are vitamins that you have to take as supplements; in other words, you should take a multi-vitamin supplement.

Vitamin B-12 is usually found only in animal proteins, and Vegans especially need to be conscious of this. Separate from a multi-vitamin, they are available as supplements that dissolve under your tongue, and others that you spray under your tongue, there are even ones you swallow. Your body stores Vitamin B-12, and it stays with you for days, so you only need to use it once or twice a week, unless blood tests show you are low in B-12.

You could ask your doctor to test your blood to see if you're low in any vitamins, like B-12, and test to see if you are low in any enzymes, like CoQ-10; they can also test you for fungus or yeast like Candita.

Vitamin C needs to be consumed on a daily basis due to the fact that it cannot be made out of foods without it (like other vitamins) and you urinate out all the Vitamin C in your system, everyday. Vitamin C should be taken on a daily basis, as a supplement, along with Vitamin E, as both are powerful antioxidants that eliminate "free radicals." Vitamin C is covered more fully in the chapter, "Natural 'cures' for cancer."

Blue green algae is a super food that has all the minerals of the ocean, which are all the minerals you need for your body; in addition, blue green algae oxygenates and repairs your cells, kills cancer cells, and is a great source of nutrition.

"Grade B" maple syrup is full of minerals. There is a "cleansing fast" that uses Grade B maple syrup as the sole source of nutrition (along with lemon juice, and cayenne pepper) for up to 30 days; as maple syrup is the sap of a tree, concentrated 50 to 100 times, it has all the minerals a tree needs. The minerals found in maple syrup are already in a state to be absorbed into cells, as the tree has special organisms living around it's smallest roots that change the minerals in the soil into usable liquid minerals.

Between blue green algae, "grade B" maple syrup, a varied diet of locally grown fruits and vegetables (in season), freshly juiced raw vegetables, and sea salt instead of rock salt, most vitamins and minerals will be present in sufficient quantities in your diet. However, an additional multivitamin and mineral supplement could be useful.

The many types of supplements include standard mineral pills (ground up rocks), chelated minerals (bound to amino acids), ionic minerals (bound to salts, in water), and colloidal minerals (reduced in size, and suspended in water). Generally, liquid minerals are more absorbable than pills, and the amount of minerals that are available to be absorbed ranges greatly; standard mineral supplement pills are generally quoted as being 3% absorbable, chelated pills around 6%, ionic liquid minerals around 10-15%, chelated liquid minerals around 30-40%, and colloidal (liquid) minerals around 50-80% absorbable. All forms of liquid minerals are available thru health and nutrition supplement stores, and many multilevel marketing groups in the United States.

Chapter 8:
Showering in filtered water

Most people know that they should drink filtered water, to avoid the chlorine, fluoride, and other toxins in the water, but did you know that you absorb 7 to 10 times more chemicals from showering, than from drinking tap water? In other words, if you don't filter your shower water, then why drink filtered water? You only address 10 - 20% of your exposure to the chemicals in tap water by drinking filtered water.

There are a variety of solutions to the problem, ranging greatly in price.

At the high end, you could buy a "whole home" water treatment system from a reputable dealer. Culligan charges around $3,000 for a, "water softener," and a, "big blue," or optional carbon tank installed "inline" before the water softener. Water softeners work by trading out dirt and chemicals for salt or potassium; you can either have a simple water softener installed along with a carbon tank, or some brands of water softener can have carbon and "KDF-55" (a form of copper/zinc) built into the tank, either way, you want "water softening," as well as "carbon," to remove chemicals. Generally, a "reverse osmosis"

(R.O.) drinking water system is sold and installed along with a water softener, they cost around $500, and last for years on "soft water" without needing a filter change.

On the low end, you can buy a, "shower filter." Shower filters install between the showerhead, and the pipe coming out of the wall; unscrew the showerhead, screw the filter onto the pipe, and then screw the showerhead back onto the filter. You can pay anywhere from $50 to $100 for a shower filter, and many are available online.

Because they are small, shower filters only reduce the chemicals in the shower water by about 90 - 95%, depending on the model, and then slowly become less effective over time as they are used. Still, a 90 - 95% reduction in chemicals from showering is a lot better than nothing, and shower filters are within everyone's price range; as they become less effective over time, you should buy extra cartridges, and replace them every few months.

If you are avoiding chlorine and fluoride in the shower water and drinking water, you should also probably avoid name brand toothpastes. All name brand toothpastes contain fluoride, while alternative brand toothpastes are available at health food stores with no fluoride. It has been suggested that the fluoride in toothpaste is capable of producing cancer in your body, and that it is possibly a toxin.

Chapter 9:
Stress and sleep

Stress has been linked to cancer, and it cannot be overlooked in a cancer recovery program. There are many ways you can remove stress, you can go out into nature, and watch animals, or even better yet, you can go to an ocean, or a lake, or a mountain, and look out over the vast blue expanse. This triggers seratonin to be released, which helps relax you.

Another great thing to do is go outside into the backyard, or to a park with your dog, or into the backyard with your cat, and just pet them, and be with them as they watch birds and squirrels; this is also a very powerful way to relax. You can also watch the fish in a fish tank, instead of watching television.

Meditation has been clinically shown to help people healing from cancer, and there are many ways to meditate; simply sitting erect and breathing is a good way to start. Try not to think; if thoughts arise, ignore them, and let them go. This simple form of meditation is actually easier out in nature, where you can sit and watch birds, and other animals.

Sleep is very important, since you heal yourself while you sleep; try to get 9 – 10 hours of sleep in the dark; turn off all the lights, and the television, draw the shades, whatever you have to do to make it dark. If you can, sleep while it's dark outside.

Chapter 10:
Limit cell phone use

Cell phones should only be used on speakerphone, and you should set them down while using them. One study showed a 240% increase in head tumors on the side of the person's head used for cell phones (usually near their ear) versus the other side of their head; and while 95% of these tumors were non-cancerous, it is still a warning sign to avoid holding cell phones to your ear. Tumors are likely associated with the electromagnetic field (EMF) generated by the cell phone.

If you hold a cell phone to your ear for around two minutes or more, you heat up all the molecules inside and outside your brain; as molecules heat up, they spin faster and get smaller.

There is a membrane at the surface of the brain called the blood-brain barrier that has holes in it a certain size to keep some things in, and some things out.

Heating molecules up spins them faster, they get smaller, and things that are not supposed to get into your brain can get in, and things that are not supposed to get out of your brain can get out.

Chapter 11:
Natural cures for cancer

The whole key to cancer fighting is in the fact that cancer cells thrive in low-oxygen-acidic-conditions, and produce lactic acid as a byproduct of the fermentation process that they use to make energy, making it more acidic inside the cell. So you can address it from either side; you can either boost the oxygen to the mitochondria in your cells, or you can balance the acidic pH condition of your body by delivering calcium to your cells that can penetrate the cell walls, and balance the pH inside the cells.

In addition to addressing the acidic-low-oxygen-conditions, there are many, "natural cures," for cancer that have been around since the 1960's, or longer, as well as new ones emerging thru scientific research, mostly overseas; and there are a number of foods that are considered as preventatives to cancer, either because they are antioxidants, or because they contain other active ingredients that repair and replace aging genes.

The work on a genetic level has progressed to the point where they should just hold a press conference, and say they've found the cure for cancer.

Scientists started looking at the human genes, and they found things that can, "turn on," or "turn off," bits of your genetic code, resulting in the cancer cells either being told to die like regular cells do, or told to digest themselves; all while not effecting the surrounding healthy cells, which allows your body to heal itself.

What is not available to purchase at your local supplement store, is available online. The website http://www.ananticancerdiet.com was set up to support this book, and has links to suppliers of the following recommended products.

Information on numbers 3 - 11 in the following list was drawn from, "Cancer Fighting Strategies," (http://www.cancerfightingstrategies.com); this is an excellent resource, with detailed information on many natural cancer treatments.

If you have been diagnosed with cancer, you might want your doctor to test you again after two or three weeks on the following list of eleven oral supplements.

Eleven cancer-fighting supplements

1) Vitamin C (shown to fight cancer with intravenous delivery).

2) Colloidal Silver (kills all bacteria, virus, fungus, and yeast, which may be an underlying cause of cancer).

3) Zeolite (activates the P21 gene that tells the cancer cells to die like normal cells).

4) CoQ-10 (shown in 1961 to be lacking in cancer patients, it helps deliver oxygen to the inside of your cells).

5) MSM (has other health benefits, but is used here mainly as a catalyst to help other substances cross into the cells).

6) Oxy-E (oxygenates your cells, which cancer hates; cancer likes a low oxygen, high acid environment).

7) Elemental pH (corrects a high acid environment in your body by delivering tiny pieces of electrically charged calcium to your cells).

8) Blue-Green Algae (repairs your mitochondria by providing replacement enzymes, also provides all the minerals needed for your body).

9) U-Fn 35% Kombu concentrate (activates a gene that tells cancer cells to digest themselves by releasing enzymes).

10) PapayaPro enzymes (papaya powder contains protease, which helps to break

down the fibrin coating of all cancerous tumors).

11) Probiotics (good intestinal bacteria, which are linked with healthy immune response).

Zeolite and U-Fn 35% Kombu concentrate should be taken in therapeutically large doses, for fighting cancer, generally three bottles per month (of each) for stage 1 cancers, and seven bottles per month (of each) for stage 4 cancers.

1) Vitamin C, as its name implies, is a "vital" "mineral" (vita-min), but for humans, it is a unique substance. Humans cannot make Vitamin C from whatever they eat; a deer makes Vitamin C out of the grass and plant shoots it eats, a lion makes Vitamin C out of the deer it eats, almost every living thing on the planet makes Vitamin C out of foods that do not contain Vitamin C, but humans have to consume foods with Vitamin C in them every day. Making this worse, we get rid of all the Vitamin C we have, on a daily basis, in our daily urine.

Linus Pauling was the only person in history to be awarded two Nobel Prizes in two different fields (without having to share them); he was awarded the Nobel Prize for Science, in 1954, and then 9 years later, the Nobel Peace Prize. He took 10 grams of Vitamin C per day to prevent colds, and he stated, quite clearly, that cancer could be cured with Vitamin C, and even co-wrote a book, "Cancer and Vitamin C", in the early 1970s. As to cancer, he advocated very high intravenous doses of Vitamin C.

2) Colloidal Silver is another natural cure for cancer. There is an oncologist (cancer specialist) who has documented that silver kills over 650 known forms of bacteria, virus, yeast and fungus; basically anything one-celled, or smaller. As to cancer, evidence points to all cancers being cured by intravenous silver therapy. This links cancer to an invasive organism (candida yeast, etc.) as the cause of the cancer, and killing this organism, "cures," your cancer.

Silver is available as an oral supplement called, "colloidal silver," and can be purchased in most health and nutrition supplement stores in America. The FDA has made the manufacturers remove all health claims, and post warnings to not use colloidal silver for more than 10 days. If you are going to use colloidal silver therapeutically for cancer treatment, and wish to exceed the FDA warning of 10 days, you should do so only under a doctor's supervision.

For the purposes of cancer treatment, there are also alternative health centers that will put colloidal silver right into your veins with an intravenous drip. As a supplement, you could always just drink some every day, which would build up a level of colloidal silver in your bloodstream anyway. Always follow colloidal silver with probiotic supplements to reestablish good intestinal bacteria.

3) "Zeolite" is a volcanic mineral that has some very impressive statistics to back it up. In a 14-month study of 65 people with mostly stage 4 cancer, Zeolite cured 51 of them, that is, over 78%. Available in liquid and powdered forms, evidence points to powders being more effective for cancer treatment, as you can take them in very large quantities, where as liquids are obviously diluted. Therapeutic dosage for fighting cancer is 3 - 7 bottles a month; 3 bottles for stage one cancers, and 7 bottles for stage four cancers. If you are fighting cancer, take Zeolite; it kills the cancer cells by activating what they call the, "P21," gene in cells, which is turned off in cancer cells, as this is normally turned on in healthy, normal cells, Zeolite only effects cancer cells, or any other cell that has had the P21 gene turned off, this tells the cells to die, like normal cells do.

4) CoQ-10 is used by the mitochondria to move oxygen around within the cells. Studies from way back in 1961 showed that most cancer patients had very low levels of CoQ-10 in their blood, reversing this "fights" cancer. Acidic conditions and low oxygen levels go hand in hand, as cancer cells use a form of low-oxygen acidic fermentation that produces more acid as a byproduct, and drives down oxygen levels further.

5) MSM (Methyl-sulfonyl-methane), a form of sulfur, may help CoQ-10 to cross thru the cell walls and get inside where it is needed; it also provides sulfur to your cells, and is said to help arthritis pain and stiffness.

6) "Oxy E" is another product that produces cellular oxygen levels sufficient to kill cancer; MSM may also help this product work better, and combined with CoQ-10, oxygenates your cells, which makes the cancer cells die.

7) Elemental pH; as everything seems to tie back to an "acidic condition," there are products that have been optimized to correct this pH imbalance, like an egg shell calcium called "Elemental pH," that you only need the tip of a teaspoon full of, to balance your pH; it is burnt at 10,000 degrees, which changes it into tiny

particles that want to cross into the cells of your body. There are many other calcium products of varying dosages, and delivery systems, read the labels at a nutrition and supplement store, or ask the clerk for the one that puts the most calcium into your cells in the best way.

8) Blue-green algae are effectively used by cancer patients, and are also, "oxygen related." In cells that have been oxygen deprived, the mitochondria are missing certain enzymes; in theory, a blue-green alga provides these enzymes for your cells to use, as replacements. Blue-green algae are also capable of balancing your pH (as cancer patients are usually very acidic), and it has been noted for its "cellular regenerative" abilities, as well as it's ability to deliver all the minerals of the ocean, which are all the minerals you need.

9) U-Fn 35% Kombu concentrate comes from "Kombu," or brown Japanese seaweed. "U-fucoidan" is the name of the active anti-cancer ingredient in Kombu; U-fucoidan has been shown to destroy cancer cells in test tubes within 72 hours, activating a gene that tells the cancer cells to digest themselves. It has been shown to be effective against a variety of cancers in human patients, ranging from stomach cancer to

leukemia, and to reduce enlarged prostate glands. Kombu is naturally very rich in U-fucoidan and should be considered as a food source, but the product listed is concentrated to 35% U-fucoidan, and like Zeolite, it should be taken in therapeutically large doses for the purpose of cancer fighting, 3 – 7 bottles per month, depending on the stage of cancer.

10) PapayaPro contains mature green papaya powder, plus Citrus Pectin, Mangosteen, and other anti-cancer ingredients. Papaya powder is an enzyme supplement that has been shown to be beneficial to your immune system, and should be taken with meals to aid digestion; papaya enzymes contain protease, which helps to break down the fibrin coating of all cancerous tumors.

11) "Probiotic" supplements are another key factor in immune response; probiotics are "beneficial" bacteria that should be living in your intestines. Some researchers claim that 70% of your immune system response is related to these organisms. Chemical exposure, as well as antibiotics kills some of these "good" intestinal bacteria, and other "bad" bacteria grow in their place. A probiotic supplement should be taken on a daily basis in pill form, as most foods (like

yogurt) either contain no cultures because they are pasteurized, or contain so few as to be of no use, since your stomach acid will kill the rest.

Many probiotic pills include from 10 to 50 different kinds of beneficial organisms (you are generally better off with a higher number). Each pill contains billions of, "live organisms," as most will die in your stomach acid before making it to their new home, in your intestines.

Chapter 12:
Making yourself younger

Science tells us that on a genetic level, we are falling apart. If you imagine the DNA "spiral staircase," the railing can fall off, and then when you make a copy of this gene, it is now different from the way the gene started out. Replacing the railing with so-called, "phytonutrients," may be able to prevent this.

Basically, brightly colored fruits and vegetables, of all colors, contain substances that are supposed to repair bits of A, C, G, or T that have fallen off your genes, so juicing is good for this, but the best way to fix this problem may be to eat blue green algae, which replaces enzymes missing from the mitochondria.

CoQ-10 has a lot of useful qualities, and may keep the ends of your genetic spiral staircase from falling apart, which is another way that copies of the genes can be made that are not like the original. MSM also helps CoQ-10 work better at delivering oxygen to your mitochondria; CoQ-10 and MSM are both included in the eleven recommended supplements in the chapter on, "natural cures," for cancer.

Giving your body all it needs is essential as well, so eat hemp seeds, blue green algae, Kombu, and coconut oil, take vitamin and mineral supplements, get exercise on a daily basis, and get 9 – 9½ hours of sleep in the dark. Drinking lots of filtered, or good quality water is also a great way to look younger, and stay healthier.

Avoiding all trans fats seems to be important to looking and actually becoming younger, even on the level of your arteries and veins. Trans fats are accused of telling your genes to switch to old person arteries, no matter what age you are. It is thought that this can be triggered by very small amounts of trans fats, like 2 grams per day; "trans fat," is another name for hydrogenated oils and partially hydrogenated oils.

Chapter 13:
Lose weight by eating more

Well, that is, more of the right foods. There are a number of people that an, "increased metabolism diet," works for. Basically, the logic goes that if you give your body all it needs, and feed it 5 times a day, then your genes tell your body to get rid of all the stored fat, because clearly, food is plentiful.

The opposite of this is the, "starvation diet," where you try to lose weight by eating less, or only once or twice a day, and you can't shed fat, this is because your body again, sees the world thru the nutrition you give it, and if you only feed yourself twice per day (skipping breakfast, for example, as in the "sumo wrestler's diet"), your body has no choice but to decide that food is scarce, and that you need to hold onto all fat reserves, in case things get worse, and you start to starve.

Your body doesn't know that you have a good job, with plenty of money for food, or enough money in the bank to eat for years; it only knows what you feed it, and how often.

All of our ancestors, within the last few thousand years, have had to survive cycles of starvation that often stretched for decades.

Holding onto fat is a survival technique that has been passed down genetically thru to today. If you understand this, then you can send a message to your genes to get rid of all stored fat, by giving yourself small amounts of food, 5 times a day.

Eating hemp seeds can also help to shed fat, since you are giving your body all the protein and essential fats it needs. Like the CRON diet in the following chapter, increased metabolism dieters should eat three tablespoon of hemp seeds, one to three times per day, so that their bodies know everything is fine with food.

Chapter 14:
Living longer lives

Additional research has given us the, "CRON," diet (Calorie Restriction with Optimal Nutrition); which basically breaks down to a 20% - 30% reduction in calories from a normal U.S. government recommended diet for adults. Adult males are typically said to need to consume 2,500 calories in a day, to stay healthy, while adult females are typically said to need to consume around 2,000 calories per day. CRON   says that adult males should consume between 1,700 - 2,000 calories per day, and adult females, between 1,300 - 1,600 calories (a 20 - 30% reduction in calories).

The reasoning goes that in lab rats, when you reduced their food by 1/3, they lived on average, twice as long as normal rats. Taken to the human level, CRON seems to contradict the "increased metabolism" diet, but they can actually work together, if you find the middle ground.

On any CRON diet, you should eat hemp seeds three times a day with meals, 3 tablespoons of hemp seeds contains about 174 calories (all of them good for you), so 3 times a day gives you 522 calories per day from hemp seeds, which provides all essential fatty acids and essential amino acids; other than blue green algae and maple syrup for minerals, and vitamin supplements, all you need is a little complex carbohydrates.

This means that you don't have to worry about getting proper nutrition; just eat 5 small meals per day; suggestions on meals are given in the following chapter.

For an adult male, try eating around 2,100 calories per day, split into 5 meals; for example: breakfast - 500 calories, brunch or a "Cliff" bar - 250 calories, lunch - 500 calories, afternoon snack - 250 calories, and dinner - 600 calories, equals a total of 2,100 calories.

For an adult woman, try 1,700 calories in a day, instead of the USRDA of 2,000 calories; for example, over 5 meals: breakfast - 400 calories, brunch or a "Luna" bar - 200 calories, lunch - 400 calories, afternoon snack - 200 calories, and dinner - 500 calories, equals a total of 1,700 calories.

With no proof in humans yet, I would guess that if 1/3 less calories makes rats live twice as long, 1/6 less might make humans live half again longer, give or take; that could mean another 30 or 40 years, for many people. Generally, the CRON diet will make someone drop between 10% and 25% of their healthy, normal, lowest adult weight.

For example, if you are an adult male, weighing 170 pounds now, and don't really have a lot of extra fat on you, CRON expects you to drop to between 130 - 155 pounds.

If you are an adult female, weighing 140 pounds now, and don't really have a lot of extra fat on you, CRON expects you to drop to between 110 - 125 pounds.

If you are overweight now, use a "calorie restricted diet with optimal nutrition," along with an "increased metabolism diet," to drop to your lowest healthy adult weight first, and then move to your CRON weight, if you wish.

Eating hemp seeds and coconut oil, as well as blue green algae, and Vitamin C and E supplements once or more per day, and a vitamin B-12 supplement once or twice a week, will add to the chances of longevity.

Getting exercise that raises and lowers your heart rate, instead of standard "cardiovascular" exercise, has also been shown to extend life, so set the inclining treadmill to have you walk up and down hills, at least, or on a stationary bike, just "sprint" for 10 or 20 seconds, and then take it easy for 30 seconds to a minute, when you're ready again, "sprint" as fast as you can until you feel your heart racing, then take it easy again.

If you can play basketball or soccer, or other sports that do this naturally, just play sports. Sprinters in training have the ideal exercise for living longer; this kind of exercise has also been shown to improve cholesterol numbers.

Meat, dairy, and eggs were a great way to avoid starvation, over the last few thousand years, and are still better than nothing if you are starving. But because they break down into more acid than vegetables, grains, and legumes, they may contribute to an overall acid state that cancer cells thrive in. So today, if you can afford to not starve, then you can make the choice to eat animal proteins, or not.

Chapter 15:
Sample Anti Cancer Diets

Breakfasts

Select one or two small portions, typically the size of the fist of the person eating. Always eat 3 tablespoons of hemp seeds with any breakfast (3 tablespoons = 174 calories).

Cold cereals with the choice of soy, rice, almond, hemp, or oat milk.

Hot cereals (oatmeal, grits, polenta, cream of wheat, etc.) with hemp seeds, coconut butter, and maple syrup; oatmeal absorbs bad cholesterol, and contains soluble fiber.

Pancakes or waffles (with coconut butter and maple syrup).

Fruit (organic, fresh, and in-season); one apple contains 4 grams of insoluble, "dietary," fiber out of the 20 you need per day.

Grapefruit, or orange juice.

Hemp-banana smoothie made with frozen banana pieces equal to one or two bananas, 3 tablespoons of hemp seeds, and rice or almond milk to barely cover; add frozen blueberries for variety.

Toast (Staff of Life aka Ezekiel bread) with coconut butter and jam, jelly, or marmalade (made without high fructose corn syrup); this kind of bread provides 2-3 grams of insoluble dietary fiber, per slice, out of the 20 grams per day we should get.

Green tea, or hot water (heated on the stove, no microwave); green tea contains ingredients with anti-cancer properties, as well as the ability to lower bad cholesterol, and restore youth. Hot water is better than cold water for healing, since you don't have to waste energy heating it up in your stomach.

Water, room temperature, since we should always drink 8 - 10 glasses of filtered water per day, this is a good time to start, if you haven't already had a glass.

Brunch

Vegetable juice, 8 - 12 oz of freshly juiced organic vegetables, carrot-beat-celery is a good base to start with, and add some of whatever other vegetables that are in season and have bright colors; if the person drinking the vegetables doesn't like the taste, add some organic fruits to the mix, like apples, melons, or whatever else is in season at the farmers market.

Always follow juice with an equal amount of room temperature, filtered water, to swish out your teeth, dilute the juice, and just because you need to drink water.

Lunches

Select one or two small portions, typically the size of the fist of the person eating. Always eat 3 tablespoons of hemp seeds with any lunch (3 tablespoons = 174 calories).

Sandwiches: avocado is a great addition to any sandwich, and provides a great protein-fat mouth feel to satisfy people missing meat and cheese sandwiches. Try avocado with lettuce, tomatoes, and sea salt on toasted Staff of Life (aka Ezekiel) bread.

Salads: made with whatever you want, no meat, cheese, or eggs though, and vinaigrette dressing.

Soups: cold or hot, anything without meat, dairy, or eggs.

Leftovers: don't microwave them.

Afternoon snacks (Green tea, other tea, hot water, or room temperature water.)

Fresh fruit: local, and in season, or dried fruits (no high fructose corn syrup added), nuts (no hydrogenated oils or high fructose corn syrup added), and dark chocolate; or a Cliff bar for men, or a Luna Bar for women; some have dairy, so check the ingredients, and avoid those.

Dinners

Select one or two small portions, typically the size of the fist of the person eating. Always eat 3 tablespoons of hemp seeds with any dinner (3 tablespoons = 174 calories).

Vegan soups, hot and cold, and Stews. A simple Vegan pea soup can be made by cooking diced onions, carrots, and celery in walnut oil at low heat for about 10 minutes in a deep pot, stir in some diced garlic for about a minute, then fill with water and a few cups of washed and sorted split peas, or lentils, add sea salt and ground black pepper; bring to a boil, then reduce to a low simmer and cook for a few hours with a cover, stirring occasionally until everything breaks down; add water if necessary; finish with soy sauce, and more sea salt and ground black pepper.

Chinese food with vegetables, mushrooms, and fried firm tofu, on rice or noodles.

Mexican food with refried beans, rice, guacamole, corn chips and salsa, or Vegan burritos, enchiladas, or tacos.

Pan fried seasoned firm tofu, mashed potatoes, and mushroom gravy, with grilled or fried vegetables.

Vegetable Pot Pie with potatoes, carrots, peas, and mushroom gravy.

Goulash and other tomato and noodle dishes

Spaghetti or gnocchi with marinara sauce, garlic bread, and salad with vinaigrette.

(For a meat substitute, slice up fresh mushrooms or crumble or slice firm tofu that was previously frozen, and fry in walnut oil on medium heat, or a combination of walnut and peanut oil on medium-high heat, with sea salt and cracked pepper, then add to any dish for continued cooking.)

Deserts

Cakes, pies, and cookies can be made with stevia instead of sugar; stevia is an indigestible substance that tastes sweet to the tongue found naturally in high amounts in bananas.

Coconut oil, aka "coconut butter," can be substituted into baked goods instead of butter or shortening, as long as you're baking at 350 degrees or lower.

Arrowroot powder, mixed in a little water, binds like an egg.

Soy, rice, almond, hemp, or oat milk can be substituted for cow's milk in baked goods recipes, though they don't act the same, and you have to experiment.

Chapter 16:
Adapting other recipes

Most people already have vegetarian family recipes, in the meals their parents and grandparents cooked in the past.

Due to necessity, most people on the planet only eat meat once or twice a week anyway, and so there are thousands of vegetarian recipes available; many people find that adapting existing family recipes is easier than learning to cook a lot of new things.

Many recipes can be adapted to Vegan by simply trading out bad proteins and fats for good ones. Between fresh and frozen tofu, and fresh and dried mushrooms of various types, almost any meat dish can be made without meat.

Dairy is a little harder to adapt, since there is actual chemistry at work; without eggs, butter, and milk, you really can't make a lot of deserts, or an omelet, but you can still bake a variety of desserts with coconut oil, and soy, rice, almond, hemp, or oat milk.

Take your favorite recipe with meat, and identify which ingredients need to go: trade butter for coconut oil, and meat for tofu and mushrooms, you'll be surprised how easy it is to make an unhealthy recipe healthy.

Whatever you know how to cook now should be the basis of healthy cooking in your house; look to family recipes, the older they are, the more likely they are to be vegetarian.

See the deserts section at the end of the previous chapter for specific substitutions in baking, like coconut butter for cow's butter, stevia for sugar, and arrowroot powder mixed in water for eggs.

Chapter 17:
Cooking with mushrooms

Get to know mushrooms; they add complex flavors to Vegan sauces and gravies. If diced to the proper size, and cooked to bring out the best flavor, they can substitute into family recipes and provide a satisfying replacement for meat. The following is a short list of some of the many commercially available mushrooms in the United States:

1) White or Brown "button" mushrooms, of all sizes, are the portabella mushroom (Italian); this is the most common mushroom in the U.S., and it can be found in every grocery store. The white ones are either kept in the dark to keep them white, or come from a mutant strain of white portabella mushroom from the 1920's in America. Brown button or table mushrooms are sometimes sold as "crimini" mushrooms; this is the unopened stage of portabella. The French call these mushrooms "champignons," and everyone has a different name for them. Portabella is a gilled mushroom, and this is where the mushroom can start to break down, and get foul, especially on older mushrooms. The button, or portabella

mushroom, is the most commonly cultivated mushroom in Europe and the United States, and can be cooked at any speed, or eaten raw; this is, in fact, the only mushroom that you might consider eating raw, and even these are probably better for you cooked; they can be cooked on low, medium, or high heat with different oils for different textures and flavors.

2) Oyster mushrooms grow on fallen trees, primarily, but can be cultivated as well; they are white, almost coral looking clusters, and while they have little mushroom caps, they don't really have gills, more like ridges to support the caps. Oyster mushrooms range around the color white, they can be off white, but it should be uniform color throughout. As the name implies, oyster mushrooms can have a taste that could be compared to mild seafood, the key is cutting them to a uniform size, and cooking them on medium to medium-low, with a little oil and salt to allow the flavors to be released.

3) Chanterelles are fairly common in the United States, and are similar to the oyster, in that they also lack true gills, and again have ridges supporting the caps, they grow on the ground in clusters, and are orange; due to their color, they

are very unmistakable in the market. These have a denser texture than oyster mushrooms, and require an even longer cook time on medium-low heat in a little oil and salt.

4) Morel mushrooms are also unmistakable; they are unique in looking like a cross between a pinecone and a sponge. Seasonally available fresh in the spring in the U.S., and available year round dried; morels are very different from other mushrooms. Science tells us that 100,000 years ago, the ancestors of the morel "mushroom" were simple one-celled yeasts, cousins to the yeasts that still make wine, beer, and hard cider today. Sometime over the last 100,000 years, they adapted to create colonies below ground like coral; from a mycelia layer a few inches below ground, hollow honeycombed shells of different sizes and thickness emerge in the spring, after rains.

Morels have a short shelf life once picked, unless they are dried immediately in a food dehydrator; they can almost have a better flavor when dried, and then reconstituted in hot water. They can be breaded, when fresh (check for bugs inside the hollow), and then fried; or, fresh or reconstituted, morels are delicious simply sliced up and sautéed with a little diced onion in some walnut oil and sea salt.

5) Porcini mushrooms (Italian) are also easy to identify in the market when fresh, as they have a pale, dense, small pored sponge under the cap, not gills. It is usually available dried, in pieces, in the stores year round. Its official name is Boletus edulis, "the delicious bolete," and it is probably the most flavorful mushroom available, short of truffles.

The flavor seems to intensify when porcinis are dried and reconstituted in hot water, and this takes about 10 minutes to an hour, depending on how they were dried and how long they were stored. Fresh or reconstituted, porcinis require the longest cook time of all the mushrooms listed to bring out their flavor; their complex earthy flavors will not come out if sautéed, browned, or caramelized.

Cook them in a little oil and salt on the lowest temperature possible, if you add diced onion after 10 minutes of cooking, the onions should only "sweat," at the temperature you have the pan, turning clear, cook for another 10 minutes, or more.

6) Truffles grow belowground, they are intensely flavored clusters, or balls, usually

available as truffle oil in the United States; truffle oil is made by cooking the truffles in oil at very low heat, to extract the flavor. Buying one $20 bottle of truffle oil will go a long way; truffle oil has an intense flavor, like liquid smoke, only a few drops are required to add a whole depth of flavor to a dish. As it could be overpowering, this is not a cooking oil, it is a flavor-adding oil; you can either add two or three drops to a stew, or gravy near the beginning of cooking, or use truffle oil as a "finishing" oil, adding a few drops near the end of cooking, or after the pan has been removed from the heat.

Basic buying and storage tips for mushrooms are:

Always inspect the mushrooms at the store, buy only firm, fresh looking mushrooms, in the case of portabella (button or opened stage), make sure they have firm gills; if you are buying larger portabellas, the gills will be black, but should not smell unpleasantly of fish, or rot. There are opposing views on eating the gills of mushrooms, some people do, and some don't; that's why the button mushrooms are so popular, as they haven't opened yet, and the gills are typically small. Even button mushrooms are sometimes opening up a bit, and again, the gills should smell clean. In the case of large, portabella style mushrooms, you can cut the stem off at the cap, and scrape out the gills with a spoon, this gives you a sort of bowl for the famous, "stuffed mushrooms."

Try to buy mushrooms the day you are going to use them, that way you don't have to store them; if you have to store mushrooms, place them in a paper bag, loosely close the bag, and refrigerate. Mushrooms degenerate quickly, and should be used within a day or two of purchase, if stored. Mushrooms should not be washed like vegetables, but instead, should just be brushed off to remove any dirt.

Chapter 18:
Cooking with tofu

There are two basic kinds of tofu: "silken" or soft tofu, and "firm" tofu. Tofu was invented by the Chinese Buddhists around a thousand years ago to provide a Vegan replacement for meat. Like good breads, it is a, "super food," that has been optimized for digestibility and nutrition. Tofu is made from soybeans, and there is a lot of evidence to support soybeans (in any form) being good for fighting cancer, good for heart health, and good for overall body health.

Silken tofu is an acquired texture raw, but is delicious as a snack with soy sauce and sesame oil. If cooked, it is still soft, and is excellent for tofu scrambles, as a replacement for scrambled eggs.

If soft (silken) tofu is frozen, then thawed, it can be sliced into one inch slices, and then fried on medium heat in walnut oil with a little sea salt until golden brown, and has a texture a little like scallops.

Firm, or sometimes "extra firm" tofu is capable of substituting into many dishes in place of meat. Slice into ¾ in pieces, and fry on medium heat in walnut oil with a little sea salt, turning to cook both sides to a golden brown.

If frozen, and then thawed, firm tofu can be literally squeezed out like a sponge, if sliced into 1 inch pieces and fried to a golden brown, it can replace chicken cutlets, if sliced into ¾ inch thick pieces, and cooked to a medium brown, it can replace thin pork cutlets, if diced into small pieces, or crumbled down, it can be browned in oil and can replace ground beef in most recipes, absorbing any flavors you give it.

When frying on medium heat, use walnut oil; when frying on medium high heat, mix a little peanut oil into the walnut oil.

Truly the Vegan's best friend, for a thousand years, tofu has been replacing meat in people's family recipes with optimized soy protein, and for only pennies a serving.

As scientific research tells us that soybeans are good for our bodies in many ways, eating tofu is a very convenient and healthy way to replace meat in your diet.

Shopping list (health food store)

Hemp seeds
Coconut oil
Peanut oil
Walnut oil
Vegan mayonnaise
Green tea
Cold Cereals
Soy, rice, almond, hemp, or oat milk
Oatmeal
Maple syrup (Grade B)
Stevia
Arrowroot powder
Sea salt
Ezekiel (Staff of Life) bread
Vinaigrette salad dressing
Salad ingredients
Avocados
Organic vegetables for juicing and cooking
Organic fruits
Rice, or other grains for cooking
Noodles
Split peas, lintels, or beans
Soy sauce
Silken tofu & firm tofu
Fresh mushrooms & dried mushrooms

Shopping list (supplement store)

Multivitamin and mineral supplement
Vitamin B-12
Vitamin C
Colloidal Silver
CoQ-10
MSM
Oxy-E (cellular oxygen booster)
Elemental pH (cellular calcium booster)
Blue green algae
Papaya Pro (papaya enzymes)
Probiotic supplement
U-Fn 35% Kombu concentrate (U-fucoidan)
Zeolite (powder)

If you're fighting cancer, Kombu concentrate and powdered Zeolite should be taken "therapeutically," at dosages 3 to 7 times what you would take as a supplement. With stage one cancers, therapeutic dosage is typically 3 bottles of 35% U-Fucoidan Kombu concentrate and 3 bottles of powdered Zeolite per month; with stage four cancers, therapeutic dosage is typically 7 bottles of 35% U-Fucoidan Kombu concentrate and 7 bottles of powdered Zeolite per month; many people see results within a few weeks.

Index

About the author

Robert Korczynski has been interested in alternative health and nutrition since the early 1990's when he was a food steward, buyer, and nutrition planner for a 15-member Vegetarian Co-op in Ann Arbor, Michigan, with about half of the meals being prepared for Vegans.

Robert currently lives in the Los Angeles area, and writes on the topics of health and Buddhism.

LaVergne, TN USA
29 November 2010
206676LV00008B/121/P